A RAND NOTE

N-2618-HHS

The Effect of a Prepaid Group Practice on Children's Medical Care Use and Health Outcomes Compared to Fee-for-Service Care

R. Burciaga Valdez

October 1989

Prepared for the
U.S. Department of Health and Human Services

RAND

PREFACE

This research was performed as part of RAND's Health Insurance Experiment under a grant from the U.S. Department of Health and Human Services. It considers how different organizing principles for providing medical care to children affect use and health outcomes. This Note uses data from Seattle to examine total expenditures on medical care, hospital and outpatient use, and the health effects arising from differential use of medical services by children in an HMO compared with fee-for-service practice.

A summary of this Note appeared in the February 1989 issue of *Pediatrics*. The report contains detailed information about the child utilization and health status analyses. Utilization results for adults and children together were reported by W. G. Manning, Jr., et al., in the *New England Journal of Medicine*, Vol. 310, June 7, 1984, pp. 1505–1510. Health status results for the adult population of the Seattle experiment were reported by J. E. Ware, Jr., et al., in *Lancet*, May 3, 1986, pp. 1017–1022, and by E. Sloss et al. in *Annals of Internal Medicine*, Vol. 106, January 1987, pp. 130–138. Results on consumer satisfaction with care were reported by A. R. Davies et al. in *Health Services Research*, Vol. 21, August 1986, pp. 430–452. These publications should be of interest to physicians and health policy analysts concerned with issues of health care financing, medical treatment, health status assessment, and the organization of medical care.

SUMMARY

Does a prepaid group practice deliver more or less care than the fee-for-service system and does the differential use of services affect health status when both serve comparable child populations with the same service benefits? To answer these questions, part of a large-scale social experiment in health care financing, the RAND Health Insurance Experiment, was devoted to comparing organization of service delivery issues.

The RAND Health Insurance Experiment was designed as a controlled trial of the effects of cost sharing and delivery organization on use of services, health status, and quality of care. In Seattle, Washington, we randomly assigned 693 children between the ages of 0 and 13 years to either a staff model health maintenance organization (HMO) or to one of several fee-for-service (FFS) insurance plans to examine differences in medical care use, expenditures, and health outcomes. All children had previously received fee-for-service care before their family was selected into the study.

Children assigned to HMO coverage were enrolled in a well-established prepaid group practice, Group Health Cooperative of Puget Sound. In this Note the fee-for-service plans are grouped into two categories: one that requires no cost sharing and those that require 25 or 95 percent cost sharing. Although the fee-for-service plans varied in the amount of cost sharing (0 to 95 percent), all children were covered for the same medical services, for either three or five years. All plans covered ambulatory and hospital care, preventive services, most dental services, and prescription drugs.

No differences in imputed total expenditures were observed for children assigned to the HMO or to any of the FFS plans. Children on cost sharing FFS plans, however, had fewer medical contacts and received fewer preventive services than those assigned to the HMO.

Despite these differences in medical care use, children on the cost sharing FFS plans were perceived (by their mothers) to be in better health overall than those assigned to the HMO. Yet, no significant differences in physiologic outcomes (e.g., visual acuity, hemoglobin level) were observed between FFS and HMO children.

The results of this experiment neither strongly support nor indict fee-for-service or prepaid care for children. Our results come from one HMO and may not apply to the

-vi-

fastest growing variant of the HMO, the Individual Practice Associations. These results, however, support the notion that no serious negative health effects exist for children receiving care in group or staff model HMOs compared with those receiving fee-for-service care.

ACKNOWLEDGMENTS

Numerous individuals made contributions to this work. I am especially indebted to Joseph Newhouse and Robert Brook for their insightful critiques of earlier versions of this work as well as their encouragement and support.

Willard Manning, John Ware, Jr., and William Rogers deserve thanks for instructing me in the finer points of statistical analysis and health status measurement. I also benefited from discussion with Emmett Keeler and Arleen Leibowitz.

I am indebted to the Group Health Cooperative of Puget Sound for agreeing to participate in the study and especially to its Director of Research during the experiment, Richard Hanschin, for his assistance and comments on this manuscript.

CONTENTS

PREFACE iii

SUMMARY v

ACKNOWLEDGMENTS vii

TABLES ix

Section

I. INTRODUCTION 1

II. METHODS 2
    Experimental Design 2
    Sample 3
    Measurement of Medical Care Use 5
    Health Status Measurement 5
    Health Status Analysis 8
    Potential Biases 10

III. RESULTS 14
    Medical Service Use 14
    Effects on Health Status of the Typical Child 14
    Health Outcomes for Children from Lower and Higher Family
        Income Levels 17

IV. DISCUSSION 22

Appendix

A. HEALTH STATUS MEASURES 25
B. ESTIMATED REGRESSION EQUATIONS 35

REFERENCES 47

TABLES

1.	Demographic and study values of children aged 0 to 13 years at enrollment, by type of insurance plan	4
2a.	Definitions of health status measures: health perceptions measures and parental worry	6
2b.	Definitions of health status measures: physiologic measures	7
3.	Health status values of children aged 0 to 13 years at enrollment, by type of insurance plan	11
4.	Distribution of children according to category of participation in experiment and plan	13
5.	Seattle children's medical service use by insurance plan	15
6.	Predicted exit values of health status measures for typical child, by measure and plan	16
7.	Predicted health outcomes for the typical child, by medical care organization	18
8.	Predicted exit values of health status measures for lower income child, by measure and plan	19
9.	Predicted exit values of health status measures for higher income child, by measure and plan	21
B.1.	Glossary of acronyms	36
B.2.	Health status values of children aged 3 to 18 years upon completion of experimental participation by insurance plan type	39
B.3.	Estimated regression model and corrected t-test values: role limitations	40
B.4.	Estimated regression model and corrected t-test values: social relations	40
B.5.	Estimated regression model and corrected t-test values: behavior problems	41
B.6.	Estimated regression model and corrected t-test values: mental health	41
B.7.	Estimated regression model and corrected t-test values: general health	42
B.8.	Estimated regression model and corrected t-test values: far vision with usual correction	42
B.9.	Estimated regression model and corrected t-test values: hearing loss	43
B.10.	Estimated regression model and corrected t-test values: fluid in middle ear	43
B.11.	Estimated regression model and corrected t-test values: anemia	44
B.12.	Estimated regression model and corrected t-test values: hay fever	44
B.13.	Estimated regression model and corrected t-test values: polio booster	45
B.14.	Estimated regression model and corrected t-test values: tetanus booster	45
B.15.	Estimated regression model and corrected t-test values: parental worry	46

I. INTRODUCTION

Since 1970 numerous policies have promoted various forms of prepaid group practices, especially health maintenance organizations (HMOs) [Falkson, 1980]. These policies have had their desired effect. Enrollment in HMOs is increasing rapidly—over 20 percent per year—and about 9 percent of the U.S. population is now enrolled in HMOs [Interstudy,1986]. Because enrollment in HMOs is popular with families with young children, it is important to assess the impact of HMO enrollment both on the use of services by children and on their health.

We previously reported expenditure results from our randomized experiment (the RAND Health Insurance Experiment). Imputed expenditures for adults and children taken together were about 28 percent lower in the HMO than in the fee-for-service system when care in both systems required no copayments by the patient [Manning et al., 1984; Manning et al., 1986]. We also found that cost sharing, if sufficiently large, could reduce expenditures in the fee-for-service system to the level of that observed in the HMO, but the resulting pattern of care was different. Relative to free fee-for-service care, cost sharing reduced both the number of ambulatory visits and the number of hospital admissions per person per year, whereas the HMO achieved its savings primarily through a 40 percent reduction in the number of hospital admissions.

We also have reported on the health effects for adults [Ware et al., 1986; Sloss et al., 1987]. We demonstrated that the typical adult who was randomly assigned to the HMO suffered no adverse health effects when compared with those adults who were randomly assigned to remain in fee-for-service care. Adults assigned to the HMO who at the beginning of the experiment were poor and ill, however, were less healthy at the experiment's end in two respects: they had a higher rate of bed days and a higher prevalence of serious symptoms than their counterparts in the fee-for-service system.

In this Note we present use, expenditure, and health results specifically for children.

II. METHODS

EXPERIMENTAL DESIGN

The Group Health Cooperative of Puget Sound, located in Seattle, Washington, was established in 1947 as a consumer cooperative staff model HMO [MacColl, 1966]. At the time of the experiment, 1976 through 1981, it served about 15 percent of the Seattle population, or around 325,000 people.

We randomly assigned some families previously receiving fee-for-service (FFS) care to Group Health Cooperative; these families are referred to as the group health experimentals (GHE) [Morris, 1979]. Other families from the same population were assigned to conventional fee-for-service health insurance plans that differed in the level of required cost sharing. Finally, we randomly sampled families already enrolled at Group Health Cooperative who otherwise met the eligibility requirements; this group is referred to as the group health controls (GHC).

The covered services were identical for children assigned to the HMO and those in the fee-for-service system. These services included acute, chronic, and preventive ambulatory care; all hospital care, mental health services, visual and auditory services, prescription drugs, and supplies; and all dental services except cosmetic orthodontia. Services of nonphysician providers such as audiologists, chiropractors, clinical psychologists, optometrists, physical therapists, and speech therapists were also covered. The group health controls maintained their usual service benefits; dental services were not included and limited vision care was provided. In fee-for-service plans, families were free to seek care from any provider.

Families in the experiment who agreed to receive medical care from Group Health Cooperative were not subject to out-of-pocket charges. Services unavailable from HMO but available in the community (e.g., dental care) were fully covered. Services available from the health maintenance organization but acquired outside the plan were reimbursed at 5 percent of charges unless the services were for emergency care or were approved referrals.

The conventional insurance plans were grouped according to the level of coinsurance or cost sharing. One-third of the children in the FFS component of the experiment received services with no out-of-pocket cost (0 percent coinsurance); this plan is referred to as the "free care plan." Another two-thirds of the children participated in plans that required copayments of either 25 or 95 percent of their medical bills. Their out-of-pocket expenditures were subject to a maximum limit based on family income that was generally $1000 per family, but was scaled down for the poor. Specifically, the limit was never more than 5, 10, or 15 percent of income—families were randomly assigned to one of these percentages— if the resulting limit was less than $1000. One of the 95 percent coinsurance plans (the individual deductible plan) was different in two respects. First, it placed a maximum per person expenditure limit of $150 or $450 per family per year for ambulatory services regardless of income. Second, inpatient services were free of any copayments. Plans requiring out-of-pocket expenditures will be referred to in this analysis as the "copay plans." Participants in these plans were grouped together because previous results suggested that their health outcomes were similar [Valdez, 1986], although their use rates differed [Leibowitz et al., 1985].

SAMPLE

Data came from 893 children (0 to 13 years old at enrollment) who, with their families, participated in the experiment that began in 1976 and ended in 1981. Families participated for either three years or five years. Thus, the children ranged in age from 3 to 18 years upon completion of the study. These children were representative of Seattle's children with a few intentional differences [Manning et al., 1984; Newhouse, 1974]. We excluded families with an annual income in the top 1 percent of Seattle's income distribution ($61,000, 1985 dollars). In addition, children in military families and institutions were excluded. Children born during the experiment were excluded from these analyses (but not from coverage by the experiment).

At enrollment the copay plans' sample consisted of 215 children, the free care plan sample consisted of 127 children, the group health experimental plan sample consisted of 351 children, and the group health control sample included 200 children (Table 1). About 75 percent of the copay plans' children, 80 percent of the free care plan participants, and 50 percent of the GHE participants were enrolled for three years. Assignment to three or five year participation was made at random for the experimental participants; control participants were all assigned to five year terms. During the experiment annual use of medical services did not differ significantly between the three- and five-year groups, so they were combined in these analyses [Manning et al., 1984].

Table 1

DEMOGRAPHIC AND STUDY VALUES OF CHILDREN AGED 0 TO 13 YEARS AT ENROLLMENT, BY TYPE OF INSURANCE PLAN(a)

	Fee-for-Service		Prepaid Group Practice	
	Copay	Free	Experimental	Control
No. of enrollees	215	127	351	200
DEMOGRAPHIC(b)				
Mean age (yr)	6.9	6.8	7.2	7.1
Gender (% male)	53	50	51	52
Race (% nonwhite)	7.5	4.0	4.3	7.5
Mean family income ($1984) (adjusted for family size)	23,364	20,677	24,686(c)	27,538(d)
Mean education of mother (yr)	12.7	12.4	12.5	13.8(d)
STUDY				
Hospitalization year before enrollment (%)	6.8	7.6	6.7	11.4
Mean no. physician visits the year before enrollment	2.8	2.8	3.1	4.7(d)
Physical screening examination taken (%)	63	51	56	43(d)
Enrollment for 3 years (%)(e)	75	82	48	0

(a) Insurance plans: fee-for service plans—0 percent copayment plan (free plan), 25 percent and 95 percent copayment plans (copay); prepaid group practice—experimentals (GHE) and controls (GHC). The control group is self-selected.
(b) For demographic data, entries include everyone with valid enrollment data.
(c) $p < 0.05$ for GHE and free plan contrast.
(d) $p < 0.05$ for GHC and GHE plan contrasts.
(e) The differences in this row are by design; the target percentages for the two fee-for-service plans were 75 percent, for the experimental plan was 50 percent, and for the control plan was 0 percent. Actual percentages differ because the target percentages applied to families, not children, and because of random refusals.

MEASUREMENT OF MEDICAL CARE USE

Data on use at Group Health Cooperative were abstracted from the HMO's records [Goldberg, 1983]. Data on fee-for-service use came from insurance claim forms filed with the experiment, which acted as the family's insurance company.

We determined the proportion of children who used any medical service or any inpatient service, the average number of admissions per child, and the total medical visits and preventive visits per child per year. We also calculated a measure of intensity of services that we constructed as follows. For admissions at Group Health Cooperative hospitals, we used the dollar figure that would have been charged had the admission been billed to a payer. For admissions at fee-for-service hospitals, we used the hospital's actual billed charges. For physician services, we derived imputed expenditures by assigning California Relative Value scale units to visits and procedures and valuing those units at the same dollar figure in both systems [Manning et al., 1984].

Preventive care was defined to include any well-child care, immunizations, screening examinations, routine physical and gynecological examinations, and visits with Papanicolaou examinations. We excluded visits for treatment of visual or hearing problems. Well care services were defined by the physcian's diagnosis, by use of certain procedure codes, or by the provider checking the preventive code box on the claim forms and the patient indicating that the reason for visit was preventive care.

In analyzing utilization data, we calculated sample means for each of the insurance plans using analysis of variance. Adjustments for children's sociodemographic characteristics did not affect any of our conclusions. We corrected all standard errors for intertemporal and intrafamily correlation.

HEALTH STATUS MEASUREMENT

We developed or adapted various health status indices to test the effect of cost sharing on health status. These indices measure four distinct dimensions of children's health: physical, mental, general perceptions, and physiologic function. In this Note we report data on 13 health status indices. Six indices describe parental assessments of either a child's health status or parental concerns (Table 2a); the remaining seven are from a medical history and screening examination of the child (Table 2b). Survey measures are more generic assessments than those obtained from a physical examination and are sensitive to a wide range of health problems and treatment benefits. For the

Table 2a

DEFINITIONS OF HEALTH STATUS MEASURES: HEALTH PERCEPTIONS MEASURES AND PARENTAL WORRY

Health Variable and Definition	Typical Item	Meaning of a High Score
ROLE LIMITATIONS(a): A dichotomous (0,1) measure that indicates whether a child can play, go to school, or take part in usual activities free of limitations resulting from poor health.	Is this child limited in the amount or kind of other activities (such as playing, helping around the house, hobbies) because of poor health?	Child is limited in role activities because of poor health.
SOCIAL RELATIONS(b): A standardized (0-10) scale that measures the quality of interpersonal interactions with significant individuals in the child's environment.	During the past 3 months, how well has this child gotten along with other children?	Child gets along with others well. Children with moderate to severe hearing problems score 0.28 points lower than those without such problems.(c)
BEHAVIOR PROBLEMS RATING(d): Standardized (0-100) scale that assesses the presence and amount of behavioral or conduct problems in the past	List of items that describe child's behavior or problems he or she sometimes has including argues a lot, likes to be alone, and temper tantrums.	Child often behaves inappropriately. Children with moderate to severe hearing problems score 1.6 points higher than those without such problems.(c)
MENTAL HEALTH RATING(e): A standardized (0-10) scale that measures anxiety, depression, and psychological well-being during the past month. A high score represents better mental health.	During the past month, did this child seem to be anxious or worried?	Child is often relaxed and cheerful. Children with moderate to severe hearing problems score 0.41 points lower than those without such problems.(c)
GENERAL HEALTH RATING(f): A standardized (0-10) scale that assesses perceptions of the child's health in the past, present, and future and susceptibility to illness. A high score represents better health.	In general, would you say this child's health is excellent, good, fair or poor?	Child is in excellent health. Children suffering from mild hay fever score 0.91 points lower than those without hay fever(g); children with moderate to severe hearing problems score 1.1 points lower than those without such problems.(c)
PARENTAL WORRY: A four-point scale measuring health-related worry.	Amount of worry in past three months 1 = Not at all 4 = A great deal	Parent worries a great deal about child's health. Children with a hearing problem score 0.36 points higher than those without hearing problems.(c)

(a) Constructed from 2 items for children under 5 years of age and 3 items for children 5 years and older.
(b) Constructed from 3 items for children 5 - 13 years old.
(c) Classification based on child with average hearing threshold level in better ear greater than 15 db."M
(d) Constructed from 14 items for children 5 - 13 years old.
(e) This battery was not administered to children younger than five years of age; it was constructed from 12 items for children under 14 years and 38 items for children 14 years or older.
(f) Constructed from 7 items for children under 14 years of age and 22 items for children 14 years and older.
(g) Classification based on parent responding yes to question about child ever having hay fever.

Table 2b

DEFINITIONS OF HEALTH STATUS MEASURES: PHYSIOLOGIC MEASURES

Health Variable and Definitions	Specific Scoring	Age Group Screened

ANEMIA STATUS: A dichotomous (0,1) indicator of low hemoglobin, adjusted for age and sex.	Defined as having anemia if hemoglobin falls below the following limits (in g/100ml of blood):
	Boys and Girls
	  6 months to 2 years 10.0
	  2 years to 12 years 11.0
	Boys only:
	  13 years to 18 years 12.0
	Girls only:
	  13 years to 18 years 11.5
		6 months to 18 years

HAY FEVER STATUS: A dichotomous (0,1) indicator of hay fever or other plant allergies.	Has this child ever had hay fever or other allergies to plants and grasses? 0 = No 1 = Yes	5 – 18 years

FUNCTIONAL FAR VISION: Visual acuity with usual correction in better eye (i.e., glasses or contacts). Measured in Snellen lines.	Visual impairment indicated if score greater than 2; 2 = 20/20
	  3 = 20/25
	  4 = 20/30.
		5 – 18 years

HEARING LOSS: A dichotomous (0,1) indicator of hearing impairment in the better ear.	Hearing impaired if average hearing threshold level in better ear (tested at 500, 1000, 2000 and 4000 Hz) is greater than 15 dB	4 – 18 years
FLUID IN MIDDLE EAR: A dichotomous (0,1) indicator of fluid in either or both middle ears.	Tympanometry results indicate effusion or probable effusion according to the following criteria: (mm H O) (Madsen units) -400 to -100 5 to 10 All -100 to 50 5.5 to 4.5 Flat or rounded -400 to -100 0 to 5 Flat or rounded 50 to 300 5.5 to 10 Flat or rounded	4 – 13 years, except those with ear surgery in past 6 months
POLIO BOOSTER: A dichotomous (0,1) indicator that polio booster received.	Since child was 4 years old, has he or she received polio booster? 0 = No 1 = Yes	5 – 13 years
TETANUS BOOSTER: A dichotomous (0,1) indicator that tetanus booster received.	Since child was 4 years old, has he or she received tetanus booster? 0 = No 1 = Yes	5 – 13 years

survey measures, the HIE relied on parental assessments for all children younger than 14 years of age and on self-reports for adolescents who were 14 to 18 years old. We designed age-appropriate questionnaires to gather information for infants and toddlers (0 to 4 years), for those in middle childhood (5 to 13 years), and for adolescents and adults (14 years and older) [Brook et al., 1979; Eisen et al., 1980].

Physiologic measures are specific to particular problems and medical interventions. Physiologic function was assessed with a medical screening examination for a random sample at enrollment (approximately 60 percent) and for all exiting participants. The multiphasic screening examination was carried out by trained paramedical personnel [Smith et al., 1978]. Different age groups were eligible for the various medical screening tests administered. The types of tests administered and the populations screened for each of the conditions are shown in Table 2b.

Health status information was collected at the beginning of the experiment (enrollment), annually during the study, and upon completing the study three or five years later (exit). The reliability and validity of the various health status indicators have been extensively reported elsewhere [Brook et al., 1979; Eisen et al., 1980; Foxman et al., 1983; Lohr et al., 1983; Rubinstein et al., 1985]. The health status indicators adopted or adapted by the HIE have been found to be appropriate for general populations, possess sufficient variability and reliability to detect differences in health status, and contain useful information about health status (App. A). Other considerations also guided the selection of medical screening examination tests, including logistics and acceptability to participants and the medical community.

HEALTH STATUS ANALYSIS

To analyze health outcomes we used ordinary least squares and logit regression methods to estimate the influence of explanatory" variables on a variety of response variables that measured health status. The regression equations were used to predict the influence of "explanatory" variables (type of insurance plan and family income) on health status at the end of the experiment. We accounted for the influence of other experimental manipulations (e.g., taking the screening examination and questionnaire form) and demographic and health characteristics (e.g., race, sex, baseline value of health) by including these variables in the estimated regression equations as well (App. B).

To facilitate interpretation of our results, we used the estimated regression equations to predict exit health status for children with a given set of enrollment characteristics. We calculated health status for three types of children in each type of insurance plan: the child participant with average values on all characteristics, as well as the typical child within the lower and upper halves of the family income distribution (1984 means of $15,982 and $36,628, respectively).

Each set of analyses contrasted predicted health outcomes for participants randomly assigned to the prepaid group practice with those for participants in the two fee-for-service insurance plans (free care plan and copay plans). Health outcomes for the group health experimental and control participants were also contrasted to evaluate differences within the prepaid group practice for those randomly assigned versus those who self-selected the plan.

We used two-tailed t-tests of significance to evaluate these contrasts. Because children in a family share their mother's tendency to consult a physician, observations from members of the same family contain less unique information than would completely independent observations. Therefore, statistical tests of predicted outcomes were corrected for correlation of the error term within each family. They were also corrected for nonconstant variance of the error term. Software was adapted from methods proposed by Huber [1967]. If a contrast was likely to occur by chance no more than 5 percent of the time (without correction for the multiple comparisons being made), the convention of labeling that result "significant" was followed. Contrasts falling short of this convention should not be ignored, however. Confidence intervals may indicate that despite statistically indiscernible differences at the conventional level, clinically and/or socially relevant differences are possible.

To address the issue of multiple comparisons, the various health outcome measures were tested together as a set using seemingly unrelated regression methods [Zellner, 1962]. This method of estimation allows us to take account of correlation among the error terms for each of the health outcome equations. Parental worry was not included in these equations, because it does not directly assess the health status of the child. An F-test for the various plan contrasts provides a test across the set of health outcomes and corrects for the multiple comparison problem.

The contrast between the GHE and the free care plan provides a comparison of differences in medical practice, because neither group faced out-of-pocket costs and both received the same benefit package. The GHE and copay plans comparison provides an assessment of the current alternatives for medical care in Seattle, i.e., two different forms of finance and practice that produce approximately similar levels of expenditure.

POTENTIAL BIASES

We examined several problems that, if present, could bias our results. First, the insurance plans offered may have been accepted by different kinds of families. Second, families may have dropped out of the various plans at different rates as a function of the members' health status. Finally, some data were missing: A few exit questionnaires were incomplete and for some participants screening examinations were not required upon enrollment. The latter missing data did not pose a threat of bias because the experimental design assured that they were missing at random across the plans.

Several strategies were used to evaluate these potential problems. First, we compared selected characteristics of the families who refused the enrollment offer with those of the families who accepted. If these groups were similar, there would be little reason to suspect bias. Second, we compared enrollment values for participants in each group. Third, we included in our regression equations the initial values of the health status variables as well as other variables known to influence health. Thus, we statistically controlled for any effect of nonrandom sample composition with respect to the explanatory variables. We did not, however, attempt recovery of health information from the few children who left the experimental sample prematurely; all results are based on values for those who completed the experiment. We imputed values for those children with missing data because they were not assigned to the enrollment screening examination and we estimated the regression equation using a method proposed by Dagenais [1971].

The problems that could potentially bias the results have negligible effects. First, offers to participate in the experiment were accepted by 75 percent of the families for the GHE, 93 percent for the free care plan, and 80 percent for the copay plans. The characteristics of families who refused and those who accepted, however, do not differ significantly [Brook et al., 1984; Ware et al., 1987]. Fewer statistically significant differences in demographic or initial health status than would be expected at random were observed for children assigned to the various plans (Table 1 and Table 3). (The group health control group was not assigned as noted above.) Indeed, the only difference

Table 3

HEALTH STATUS VALUES OF CHILDREN AGED 0 TO 13 YEARS AT ENROLLMENT, BY TYPE OF INSURANCE PLAN(a)(b)

	Fee-for-Service		Prepaid Group Practice	
	Copay	Free	Experimental	Control
Role limitations (% limited)	4.7	4.0	5.0	2.5
Mean social relations (0-10 scale)	5.1	5.1	5.2	5.1
Mean mental health rating (0-10 scale)	5.9	5.9	5.9	5.8
Mean general health rating (0-10 scale)	6.1	5.9	5.9	5.7
Anemia (% with low hemoglobin)	5.4	6.7	2.7	2.4
Hay fever (% bothered by plant allergies)	9.5	15.2	8.1	19.1(c)
Vision, corrected (mean in Snellen lines)	3.2	3.3	2.8	2.9
Hearing loss (% with hearing impairment)	6.2	5.0	3.5	6.6
Fluid in middle ear (% with suspected effusion)	22.4	27.0	14.5	19.0(c)
Polio booster (% with booster)	89.6	90.9	92.3	93.7
Tetanus booster (% with booster)	87.6	85.7	89.8	93.0
Parental worry (1-4 scale)	1.6	1.6	1.8	1.7

(a) Insurance plans: fee-for service plans--0 percent copayment plan (free), 25 percent and 95 percent copayment plans (copay); prepaid group practice--experimental (GHE) and control (GHC). The control group is self-selected.
(b) For physiologic data, the mean score excludes children not assigned to an initial screening examination.
(c) p < 0.05 for GHC and GHE plan contrasts.

observed was that the GHE group had a higher mean family income (adjusted for family size) than did the free care plan group. Family income was included as a covariate in our models to control for this imbalance.

Attrition from the experimental portion of this study was low. Excluding the group health controls, 96 percent of the children who participated completed their term in the experiment (Table 4). Among those randomly assigned to an insurance plan, children on the free care plan were the least likely to leave the experiment early, whereas the children on the copay plans were the most likely not to complete as scheduled. Although the copay plan participants were more likely not to complete the experiment than the GHE participants, this difference was not statistically significant. Using a Weibull survival model to adjust for time at risk, Manning and colleagues [1986] found no significant differences in loss rates among the GHE and FFS plans. For several reasons, the children in the control group at Group Health Cooperative were the most likely to leave the study before their term expired: (1) Some children were terminated when their family lost eligibility for Group Health Cooperative; this included some from families in which the parent changed jobs and the new employer did not offer Group Health Cooperative, and all who moved out of the area; (2) they were all enrolled for five years and hence had greater exposure to the risk of attrition.

Table 4

DISTRIBUTION OF CHILDREN ACCORDING TO CATEGORY OF PARTICIPATION IN EXPERIMENT AND PLAN

Category of Participation	Fee-for-Service				Prepaid Group Practice			
	Copay		Free		Experimental		Control	
	No.	%	No.	%	No.	%	No.	%
Total enrolled	215	100	127	100	351	100	200	100
Completed study	191	88.8	124	97.6	329	93.7	128	64
Voluntarily left study early	22	10.2	0	0	14	4.0	24	12
Terminated from study	1	0.5	3	2.4	8	2.3	48	24(a)
Died	1	0.5	0	0	0	0	0	0

(a) Includes children who lost eligibility for Group Health Cooperative, typically because their parent changed employers, and those whose families moved from the Seattle area. Such children were not terminated in the other three plans. In the case of the experimental group, a family that moved from the area was changed to the free plan for the duration of the experiment.

III. RESULTS

MEDICAL SERVICE USE

Imputed expenditures for children were similar in GHE and the fee-for-service plans but they were 41 percent lower than GHC (Table 5). The mean for the GHC plan was inflated by several very expensive hospitalizations as is reflected in the large standard error. Data pertaining to admissions and visits, to which we now turn, are less subject to sampling error than imputed expenditures.

The service mix in the various plans differs considerably. GHE children were less likely to be admitted to the hospital ($p < .05$) but more likely to have an office visit than children in the free care plan. The rate of hospital admissions among GHE children is about half that of those in the free care plan ($p < .10$), whereas visit rates are about 21 percent higher ($p < .10$).

The GHE children are also more likely to have contact with medical providers than children on the copay plans ($p < .01$). Hospital admission rates for the GHE children are about 17 percent lower than those on the copay plans, whereas visit rates are about 50 percent higher. Preventive visit rates for the GHE children are 40 percent higher than those on the copay plans ($p < .01$).

Differences between the group health experimentals and controls suggest a greater propensity of the control children to use medical services ($p < .01$). The control children have a 65 percent higher rate of hospital admissions and a 27 percent higher visit rate than the GHE children. Little difference is observed in the use of preventive care services for the two group health plans and the free fee-for service plan.

EFFECTS ON HEALTH STATUS OF THE TYPICAL CHILD

When we contrast the individual health outcomes of all children on the free fee-for-service plan with those in GHE, we find no statistically significant differences (Table 6). Two results approaching statistical significance—corrected vision and general health perceptions—show better outcomes on the free fee-for-service plan. Although five out of seven physiologic function measures favor the GHE, this trend was insignificant. Children on the free fee-for-service plan are in no better or worse health than the GHE children at the end of the experiment, judging by all health status measures evaluated

Table 5

SEATTLE CHILDREN'S MEDICAL SERVICE USE, BY INSURANCE PLAN(a)

(Standard error in parentheses)

Plan	Percent Using Inpatient or Outpatient Service in Year	Percent with One or More Hospitalizations in Year	Imputed Annual Expenditure per Child (1983 $)(b)	Admission Rate/100 Children(c)	Face to-Face Visits per Child(d)	Mental Health Visits per Child(e)	Preventive Visits per Child(f)
FEE-FOR-SERVICE							
Copay	74.3 (2.89)	4.18 (.974)	197 (32.4)	4.49 (1.10)	3.24 (.398)	.13 (.068)	.36 (.035)
95% Copay	71.4 (5.16)	2.82 (1.18)	124 (20.5)	3.29 (1.53)	2.36 (.366)	.277 (.189)	.286 (.053)
25% Copay	77.0 (4.87)	4.78 (2.10)	241 (79.0)	5.22 (2.37)	2.94 (.443)	.02 (.01)	.41 (.066)
ID	74.4 (4.82)	4.93 (1.49)	225 (42.0)	4.93 (1.49)	4.50 (1.05)	.0936 (.0865)	.336 (.047)
Free	83.3 (3.02)	6.55 (1.33)	228 (25.9)	6.85 (1.49)	3.24 (.276)	.14 (.074)	.46 (.061)
PREPAID GROUP PRACTICE							
Experimental (GHE)	84.8 (2.03)	3.38 (.564)	227 (18.5)	3.72 (.635)	3.91 (.239)	.07 (.028)	.50 (.027)
Control (GHC)	93.3 (1.13)	4.03 (.820)	382 (92.1)	6.12 (1.70)	4.96 (.293)	.09 (.035)	.56 (.033)
DIFFERENCE							
GHE minus free	1.5	-3.17(g)	-1	-3.10(h)	0.67(h)	-0.07	.04
GHE minus copay	10.5(i)	-0.80	30	-.77	0.67	-0.05	.14(i)
GHE minus GHC	-8.5(i)	-0.65	-155(h)	-2.40	-1.05(i)	-0.02	-.06

(a) Insurance plans: fee-for-service--25 percent and 95 percent copayment plans (copay), individual deductible (ID), 0 percent copayment plan (free); prepaid group practice--experimentals (GHE) and controls (GHC). The control group is self-selected.
(b) Values include both in-plan and out-of-plan use by prepaid group practice participants.
(c) A count of all continuous periods of inpatient care.
(d) Includes all visits with face-to-face contact with health providers for which a separate charge would have been made in fee-for-service. Excludes radiology, pathology, pre- and postoperative, speech therapy, psychotherapy, dental, chiropractic, Christian Science healer, and telephone visits.
(e) Includes psychotherapy and psychiatric visits.
(f) Includes well-child care, immunizations, screening examinations, routine physical and gynecological examinations, and visits with Pap smears (other than for cancer). Excludes vision and hearing treatment visits.
(g) p < 0.05.
(h) p < 0.10.
(i) p < 0.01.

Table 6

PREDICTED EXIT VALUES OF HEALTH STATUS MEASURES FOR TYPICAL CHILD,(a) BY MEASURE AND PLAN(b)

Health Status Measure	Fee-for-Service		Prepaid Group Practice Experimental	Difference: Free − GHE(c)	Difference: Copay − GHE(c)
	Copay	Free			
HEALTH PERCEPTIONS					
Role limitations (%)	2.8	2.5	1.9	0.6 (−2.6, 3.8)(c)	0.9 (−2.6, 4.4)
Social relations(d)	8.23	8.33	8.52	−0.2 (−.65, .27)	−0.3 (−.68, 0.1)
Behavior problems(e)	15.6	17.0	17.6	−0.6 (−3.4, 2.2)	−2.0 (−4.2, 0.28)(f)
Mental health(d)	5.70	5.73	5.61	0.1 (−.23, .47)	0.4 (−.2, .38)
General health(d)	5.72	5.70	5.33	0.4 (−.02, .76)(f)	0.4 (.08, .7)(g)
PHYSIOLOGIC MEASURES					
Vision, corrected(h)	2.7	2.3	2.6	−0.3 (−.57, −.01)(f)	0.1 (−.07, .43)
Hearing (%)	5.6	7.3	4.3	3.0 (−3.0, 9.0)	1.3 (−3.3, 5.9)
Middle ear fluid (%)	39.2	42.6	28.7	13.9 (−4.5, 32.3)	10.5 (−3.4, 24.4)
Anemia (%)	3.4	0.9	0.8	0.1 (−1.9, 2.1)	2.6 (−.32, 5.52)(f)
Hay fever (%)	17.1	16.2	18.4	−2.2 (−12.9, 8.5)	−1.3 (−10.8, 8.2)
Polio booster (%)	95.9	95.5	97.7	2.2 (−4.9, 9.3)	1.8 (−3.2, 6.8)
Tetanus booster (%)	95.3	87.5	96.9	9.4 (−2.4, 21.2)	1.6 (−4.2, 7.4)
PARENTAL CONCERN					
Parental worry(i)	1.6	1.4	1.6	0.2 (.02, .38)(g)	0 (−.13, .17)

(a) Sample sizes across measures are dissimilar because the number of children included in each health status analysis differs because of age restrictions or missing data.
(b) Insurance plans: fee-for-service--25 percent and 95 percent copayment plans (copay), 0 percent copayment plan (free); prepaid group practice--experimentals (GHE).
(c) 95 percent confidence intervals in parentheses; approximate confidence intervals for dichotomous indicator variables.
(d) 0-10 scale; a higher value denotes better health.
(e) 0-100 scale; a higher value denotes poorer health.
(f) p <.10.
(g) p <.05.
(h) In Snellen line values 2 = 20/20, 3 = 20/25, 4 = 20/30.
(i) Four-point scale--4 = a great deal, 3 = somewhat, 2 = a little, 1 = not at all.

together. Parents, however, are less worried about their children's health on the free care plan than are parents assigned to the HMO ($p < .05$).

On the basis of our best measure of overall health status, the general health rating index, parents of children on the copay plans rated their children's health more favorably than those enrolled in GHE ($p < .05$). Children on the copay plans were also rated in better mental health based on the behavior problems index but were more likely to suffer from anemia than children in GHE. No other differences approached statistical significance, despite the apparent trend for children on the copay plans to consistently do worse on the physiologic health status assessments when compared with those children assigned to the HMO. Six out of seven physiologic assessments show better outcomes for children on GHE, but only one of these, anemia, approached statistical significance. A test of the set of health status measures indicates that children on the copay plans are in better health ($p < .01$) than were the GHE children. This result is driven largely by the difference at the experiment's end in general health rating.

Examining results for the group health control children we find they are less likely to suffer from middle ear disease ($p < .05$) but more likely to suffer from uncorrected vision problems ($p < .05$) than children randomly assigned to Group Health Cooperative. (Table 7). When we evaluate the two groups on the entire set of outcomes together, differences in health status are not significant. Parents in the control group, however, express less worry about their child's health than those who were assigned to Group Health Cooperative.

HEALTH OUTCOMES FOR CHILDREN FROM LOWER AND HIGHER FAMILY INCOME LEVELS

For a subset of our measures the sample was large enough to test for differences by plan among lower and higher income children. No statistically significant differences were observed for lower income children participating in GHE compared with children in the free care plan (Table 8). Two of three health perceptions measures and two of four physiologic measures favored the free care plan. Low income parents, however, expressed less worry about their children on the free care plan.

On the basis of the general health rating index, lower income children on the copay plans were judged in better health than children in GHE. Two of three health perceptions measures favor the copay plans but three of four physiologic assessments

Table 7

PREDICTED HEALTH OUTCOMES FOR THE TYPICAL CHILD,(a) BY MEDICAL CARE ORGANIZATION(b)

Health Status Measures	Prepaid Group Practice $\bar{M}$		Control	Difference: GHC - GHE(c)	
	Experimental		Control		
HEALTH PERCEPTIONS					
Role limitations (%)	1.9		2.9	1.0	(-2.5, 4.5)
Social relations(d)	8.52		8.26	-0.26	(-.69, .17)
Behavior problems(e)	17.5		16.8	-0.7	(-3.8, 2.3)
Mental health(d)	5.61		5.64	0.03	(-.34, .40)
General health(d)	5.33		5.47	0.14	(-.27, .55)
PHYSIOLOGIC MEASURES					
Vision, corrected(f)	2.6		3.0	0.4	(.13, .67)(g)
Hearing (%)	4.5		5.5	1.0	(-4.3, 6.3)
Middle ear fluid (%)	27.9		14.3	-13.6	(-26.9, -0.3)(g)
Anemia (%)	0.8		1.4	0.6	(-2.3, 3.6)
Hay fever (%)	18.7		14.9	-3.8	(-15.6, 8.0)
Polio booster (%)	97.4		97.9	0.5	(-5.8, 6.8)
Tetanus booster (%)	96.9		98.4	1.5	(-3.8, 6.8)
PARENTAL CONCERN					
Parental worry(h)	1.6		1.4	-0.2	(-.41, -.01)(g)

(a) Sample sizes across measures are dissimilar because the number of children included in each health status analysis differs because of age restrictions or missing data.
(b) Insurance plans: Group Health Cooperative, experimentals (GHE), Group Health Cooperative, Controls (GHC). Control group is self-selected. Differences in predicted GHE scores for Table 6 and Table 7 are due to differences in modeling the fee-for-service plans.
(c) 95 percent confidence intervals in parentheses; approximate confidence intervals for dichotomous indicator variables.
(d) 0-10 scale; a higher value denotes better health.
(e) 0-100 scale; a higher value denotes poorer health.
(f) In Snellen line values 2 = 20/20, 3 = 20/25, 4 = 20/30.
(g) $p < 0.05$.
(h) Four-point scale - 4 = a great deal, 3 = somewhat, 2 = a little, 1 = not at all.

Table 8

PREDICTED EXIT VALUES OF HEALTH STATUS MEASURES FOR LOWER INCOME CHILD,(a)
BY MEASURE AND PLAN (b)
(Bottom 50% of family income distribution)

Health Status Measures	Fee-for-Service Copay	Fee-for-Service Free	Prepaid Group Practice Experimental	Difference: Free-GHE(c)		Difference: Copay-GHE(c)	
HEALTH PERCEPTIONS							
Mental health(d)	5.91	5.54	5.53	.01	(-.50, .52)	.38	(-.07, .83)(e)
General health(d)	5.84	5.42	5.24	.18	(-.35, .71)	.60	(.13, 1.1)(f)
PHYSIOLOGIC MEASURES							
Vision, corrected(g)	3.1	2.6	2.9	-.3	(-0.62, .04)(e)	.2	(-.13, .45)
Hearing (%)	8.6	6.3	5.3	-1.0	(-6.3, 8.3)	3.3	(-4.2, 10.8)
Middle ear fluid (%)	38.1	43.2	29.9	13.3	(-8.1, 34.7)	8.2	(-8.7, 25.1)
Hay fever (%)	13.1	14.1	15.8	-1.7	(-14.6, 11.2)	-2.7	(-14.3, 8.9)
PARENTAL CONCERN							
Parental worry(h)	1.6	1.4	1.6	.2	(-.05, .43)	0	(-.22, .22)

(a) Sample sizes across measures are dissimilar because the number of children included in each health status analysis differs because of age restrictions or missing data.
(b) Insurance plans: fee-for-service--25 percent and 95 percent copayment plans (copay), 0 percent copayment plan (free); prepaid group practice--experimentals (GHE).
(c) 95 percent confidence intervals in parentheses; approximate confidence intervals for dichotomous indicator variables.
(d) 0-10 scale; a higher value denotes better health.
(e) $p < 0.10$.
(f) $p < 0.05$.
(g) In Snellen line values 2 = 20/20, 3 = 20/25, 4 = 20/30.
(h) Four-point scale - 4 = a great deal, 3 = somewhat, 2 = a little, 1 = not at all.

favor GHE. No statistically significant physiologic differences, however, were observed. Nor were differences in parental worry observed.

No statistically significant differences were observed for fee-for-service children from higher income families in any contrasts with GHE participants (Table 9). Two of three health perceptions measures and two of four physiologic assessments showed better health outcomes for free care plan children than GHE children. Parents of free care plan participants also expressed less worry about their child's health.

Few differences in health outcomes were observed for higher income children participating in GHE rather than copay plans (Table 9). None of these differences were statistically significant. Two of three health perceptions measures and two of four physiologic assessments favored the GHE. Parents did not express a difference in the amount of worry they experience as a result of their child's health.

Table 9

PREDICTED EXIT VALUES OF HEALTH STATUS MEASURES FOR HIGHER INCOME CHILD,(a) BY MEASURE AND PLAN(b)
(Top 50% of family income)

Health Status Measures	Fee-for-Service Copay	Fee-for-Service Free	Prepaid Group Practice Experimental	Difference: Free – GHE(c)	Difference: Copay – GHE(c)
HEALTH PERCEPTIONS					
Mental health(d)	5.51	5.82	5.62	.2 (-.31, .71)	-.11 (-.52, .3)
General health(d)	5.56	5.89	5.36	.53 (-.04, 1.1)	.2 (-.25, .65)
PHYSIOLOGIC MEASURES					
Vision, corrected(e)	2.8	2.4	2.7	-.29 (-.62, .04)(f)	.1 (-.13, .45)
Hearing (%)	2.8	9.2	3.6	-5.6 (-3.8, 15)	-.8 (-5.3, 3.7)
Middle ear fluid (%)	39.1	45.9	25.4	20.5 (-4, 45)	13.7 (-5.7, 33.1)
Hay fever (%)	23.4	18.9	23.9	-5.0 (-12.8, 22.8)	-0.5 (-16, 15)
PARENTAL CONCERN					
Parental worry(g)	1.6	1.4	1.6	-.2 (-.06, .52)	0 (-.24, .26)

(a) Sample sizes across measures are dissimilar because the number of children included in each health status analysis differs because of age restrictions or missing data.
(b) Insurance plans: fee-for-service--25 percent and 95 percent copayment plans (copay), 0 percent copayment plan (free); prepaid group practice--experimentals (GHE).
(c) 95 percent confidence intervals in parentheses; approximate confidence intervals for dichotomous indicator variables.
(d) 0-10 scale; a higher value denotes better health.
(e) In Snellen line values 2 = 20/20, 3 = 20/25, 4 = 20/30.
(f) p < 0.10
(g) Four-point scale - 4 = a great deal, 3 = somewhat, 2 = a little, 1 = not at all.

IV. DISCUSSION

The results from our randomized controlled trial in one well established staff model prepaid group practice permit us to answer three questions. First, when care is free (i.e., requires no out-of-pocket expenditures at point of service) for both fee-for-service and HMO care, do use of services and health outcomes differ? Second, when families receiving fee-for-service care must share in the financial burden of the medical bill (i.e., have cost sharing in the insurance plan), do children in the HMO use a different mix of services and do their health outcomes differ? Third, are there any differences in service use and health outcomes for children assigned to an HMO and those whose families chose to enroll in an HMO?

The first two questions were evaluated by contrasting service use and health outcomes of children randomly assigned to an HMO or to fee-for-service insurance plans. To answer the last question, we compared use and health outcomes for children randomly assigned to Group Health Cooperative of Puget Sound with a group of children whose families were already members of the HMO.

We found that for the typical child, general health perceptions appeared better for those receiving fee-for-service care than for children assigned to the HMO. No other significant health effects were observed. Parents on the free care plan, however, also expressed less worry about their child's health than parents at the HMO. All these effects tended to be found in both high and low income groups.

The general health rating index is our best overall measure of health status. The mean difference in general health rating favoring fee-for-service care represents an effect about half the size of the perceived impact on a child's overall health of suffering from mild to moderate hay fever or about a third of the impact of moderate hearing problems on health. The 0.4 point difference we observed in plan comparisons represents about a fifth of a standard deviation in the general health rating. Thus, this statistically significant difference represents a small health effect. This adverse effect on perceived health could result from the 21 percent higher visit rate at group health [Diehr et al., 1979].

The absence of significant differences on the other survey measures is not due to poor precision because the confidence intervals for contrasts do not include differences of clinical importance. In contrast to the survey measures, many of the contrasts for the physiologic measures do have wide confidence intervals. Some of these differences would be clinically meaningful. For example, the difference in visual acuity between GHE and the free care plan groups could be as large as half a Snellen line better on the free care plan, whereas the difference in the proportion suffering from anemia could be 6 percent higher and fluid in the middle ear could be 24 percent higher on the copay plans compared with those measures for children on the GHE plan.

Given the modest health effects that we observed, the debate about the effects of prepaid group practice must focus on the use and expenditure results. Unlike our previous findings for adults and children combined, a reduction in imputed expenditures was not observed for children using the HMO. Although Group Health Cooperative children had a 46 percent lower hospital admission rate than children on the free care plan, this effect is offset by a 21 percent higher outpatient visit rate. The effect on expenditure of this large percentage reduction in hospital admissions is mitigated by two factors; when compared with similar measures for adults: (1) The absolute level of hospital admissions among children is sufficiently low that the 46 percent reduction represents only three admissions per 100 children per year; and (2) children's hospitalizations are inexpensive compared with their ambulatory care.

Compared with insurance plans having moderate coinsurance and deductible requirements, no appreciable savings from HMO participation by children was observed. Cost sharing plans, however, reduce imputed expenditures by reducing both medical contacts and inpatient care relative to plans with no copayment requirements. Children received more preventive services from the HMO than with cost sharing plans, but the difference was small relative to the free care plan, suggesting that cost sharing is the major factor deterring use of preventive services.

The patterns of use and modest health effects we observed may also reflect differences in the type of health professionals who are providing services to children. Numerous studies suggest that general/family practitioners treat children differently than do pediatricians [Hoekelman et al., 1984; Smith-Staruch et al., 1984]. Many HMOs have relied on nurse practitioners extensively to provide care to children. Group Health Cooperative of Puget Sound is no exception. Most children in Group Health Cooperative receive their primary care either from a family practice physician or a pediatric nurse practitioner. Nurse practitioners are supervised by a pediatrician. Among our fee-for-service children 16 years and younger, 62 percent received care from a specialist, 80 percent of whom received services from pediatricians [Marquis, 1984]. In spite of this level of specialist use by the fee-for-service children, they were not physiologically better off. Their parents, however, were less worried and rated their children's overall health higher than did parents of children assigned to the HMO.

Interpreting the differences between the group health experimental and control groups requires considerable caution because of the influence of self-selection, differential attrition, and differences in plan coverage. The vision effect favoring the experimentals undoubtedly results from plan differences in benefits. The experimental group children were fully covered for vision services whereas the controls were not. But the effect on middle ear disease and on parental worry may reflect the control group's preference for and mastery of the HMO system. Children in families assigned to Group Health Cooperative used fewer medical services, both outpatient visits and hospital admissions, than children in families who enrolled at Group Health Cooperative voluntarily (control group). This differential use of services suggests that families electing services from Group Health Cooperative have children who are disproportionately high users of medical care or that the families have a greater ability to make use of resources at Group Health Cooperative. Health status does not seem to explain the difference given their overall positive health status as we measured it.

Our results support the hypothesis that no serious negative health effects exist for children receiving care in the staff model prepaid group practice compared with those receiving fee-for-service care. Although children in fee-for-service care are perceived to be in better health by their parents, no physiologic differences were noted when we compared those receiving fee-for-service care with those assigned to the HMO. Our results, however, come from one staff model HMO and thus do not apply to the fastest growing variant of the HMO, the Individual Practice Associations.

Appendix A

HEALTH STATUS MEASURES

Five conditions (anemia, hay fever, fluid in the middle ear, hearing loss, and visual acuity) provide physiologic information about children in the experiment. (Additional physiologic information was collected on the following conditions: cancer, convulsions, dental conditions, bedwetting, growth and development disorders, lead poisoning, and urinary tract infections. Data on dental conditions, oral health behavior, and growth and development are the subjects of forthcoming reports. The other conditions occurred were too infrequent to provide reliable information.) The criteria used to evaluate each condition can be found in Table 1. These conditions were selected because they can be readily detected, are fairly prevalent, are amenable to medical treatment, and they have important adverse effects if left unattended.

ANEMIA

Anemia is not a disease in itself, but like fever provides a signal that a problem exists. Anemia refers to an abnormally low level of hemoglobin in the blood. It is the hemoglobin in the blood cells that transports oxygen to all parts of the body. A low level of hemoglobin can occur for a variety of reasons: loss of blood, insufficient supplies of iron or other nutrients needed to make hemoglobin, destruction of red blood cells within the body, or when disease prevents the body from replacing hemoglobin.

The reported prevalence of anemia varies widely. Using a hemoglobin concentration of 10.0 g/100 ml, the reported prevalence of anemia in children 6 months to 10 years ranges from 0.1 to 24.0 percent [Kessner and Kalk, 1973; Dutton and Silber, 1980; Dallman, 1981; and CDC, 1981]. Investigators have shown that anemia is strongly associated with a variety of environmental and family characteristics reflecting socioeconomic factors including dietary habits, income, and race [Lanzkowsky, 1974; and Dutton, 1979].

Anemia produces few symptoms unless it is severe (less than 10.0 g/100 ml). The symptoms of anemia are fatigue, shortness of breath, dizziness, and palpitations.

The most common childhood forms of anemia are associated with having smaller than normal blood cells: iron deficiency anemia or thalassemia minor [Rudolph, 1977]. The proportion of anemia in the general population caused by iron deficiency exceeds that associated with other more unusual conditions [Dallman, 1981]. Therefore, any low hemoglobin found in a general population survey such as the HIE is likely due to iron-deficiency rather than chronic disease.

We used results from a blood test from the medical screening examination to assess whether a child suffered from anemia [Foxman et al., 1983]. Blood was drawn from children 6 months and older. A finger prick was used for children younger than a year. Blood samples were analyzed on an automated Coulter Model S for hemoglobin, hematocrit, red blood cell count, mean cell volume, mean cell hemoglobin, and mean cell hemoglobin concentration. Serum iron and total iron binding capacity were assessed for children whose hemoglobin level fell below normal limits at exit. Reference standards for hemoglobin based on values obtained with electronic counters on large healthy populations were adopted for use in the HIE with the following change: The lower levels of normal hemoglobin were defined as 0.5 g/100 ml lower than the reference levels to allow for the effect of diurnal variation in hemoglobin concentration. Diurnal variations as great as 15 percent have been reported in the literature [Dacie and Lewis, 1975]. All blood samples were drawn after 11:00 a.m., and half were drawn in the evening hours. Thus, hemoglobin values would be expected to be systematically lower than values from other studies in which blood samples were drawn earlier in the day.

A child (6 months to 18 years) is defined as having anemia if his hemoglobin level fell below the following limits (grams per 100 ml of blood):

Both boys and girls:	6 months to 2 years	10.0
	2 years to 12 years	11.0
Boys only:	13 years to 18 years	12.0
Girls only:	13 years to 18 years	11.5

Two girls pregnant at the time of the screening examination were excluded from the anemia analyses.

HAY FEVER AND OTHER PLANT ALLERGIES

A noninfectious inflammatory disease of the nasal passages, hay fever or allergic rhinitis is characterized by a variety of symptoms including congestion, hypersecretion, sneezing, and itchy eyes, nose, and throat. The intensity of these symptoms varies from day to day.

Hay fever like asthma may be caused by allergic or nonallergic factors. Some of the allergens suspected of causing hay fever include: mold spores, pollens, and animal dander. Nonallergic hay fever may be the result of infections or psychosomatic processes.

Hay fever affects children either on a seasonal basis or perennially. Seasonal hay fevers are very likely allergin induced and appear only when particular allergens are present in the air. Children with perennial hay fever experience symptoms throughout the year. Constant contact with animal dander or molds or psychological distress may cause these symptoms.

The current prevalence of asthma and hay fever is estimated to be between 3 and 4 percent [NCHS, 1973a]. The cumulative prevalence for hay fever was estimated as 4.6 percent for children ages 6 to 11 and 9.2 percent for ages 12 to 17 [NCHS, 1973b]. Judging from results from the National Ambulatory Medical Care Survey of 1977, for persons of all ages, hay fever was the seventh most frequently rendered principal diagnosis for physician office visits, which accounts for 2 percent of all visits [NCHS, 1980].

Depending on the physician's definition of hay fever's minimal symptoms, a child may be labeled as having hay fever and thus may or may not be tested for an allergic cause. If the parent or child does not report or deemphasizes the symptoms when visiting the physician (or does not seek care), the disease will likely be underdiagnosed or undiagnosed.

Treatment for hay fever includes both specific and nonspecific modes. Specific modes attempt to avoid, eliminate, or immunize against a particular allergen. Nonspecific modes include the use of antihistamines, decongestants, or combinations of these two drugs. Therapies that are applied directly to the nasal mucosa should be used only on a temporary basis. If used too long or too often, they eventually irritate the mucosa and cause the symptoms they were intended to prevent.

All methods for diagnosing hay fever except the medical history were considered either impractical or too expensive for a general population survey. Thus, the HIE used a self-administered medical history questionnaire to obtain information about the presence of hay fever and other plant allergies [Beck et al., 1983]. Broder et al. [1974] showed that questionnaire responses, when compared to physician diagnosis of hay fever, could adequately discriminate between those who had hay fever, and those who did not.

VISION IMPAIRMENT

Vision impairment among children may be manifested as diminished acuity or misalignment of the eyes. These conditions may arise because of the shape of the eye, ocular muscle imbalance, suppressed vision in one eye, or congenital problems. The HIE concentrated on detecting problems of visual acuity. Because a child's eye continues to grow until early puberty, there is no universal agreement as to what level of diminished acuity constitutes a true impairment at a given age.

Numerous sources of data provide evidence that vision impairment is one of the most prevalent conditions among children in the United States. Kessner et al. [1974] found that 28 percent of children in a general population had some type of vision problem. Fully a fifth of the children surveyed had poor far-vision acuity with their corrective lenses. The National Center for Health Statistics has conducted three surveys in which vision problems were assessed: 1963–1965 (for children 6 to 11 years old), 1966 to 1967 (for children 12 to 17 years old), and 1971 to 1972 (children of all ages). Reporting levels of acuity for the better eye, the earliest study found that 38 percent of children between the ages of 6 and 11 had natural distance acuity of their better eye worse than 20/20; 20 percent had acuity of 20/30 or worse [NCHS, 1970a]. The second survey (1966 to 1967) found that among the older children 43 percent were unable to achieve 20/20 far vision acuity with one or both eyes while using their available corrective lenses during testing [NCHS, 1974]. In the most recent NCHS study (1971–1972), of children 6 to 11 years old, 27.5 percent had vision worse than 20/20 in their better eye. Among youths 12 to 17 years old, 17 percent were unable to test 20/20 far vision in their better eyes [NCHS, 1977].

Acuity deficits have the capacity to affect a child's learning abilities and his social and psychological development [NSPB, 1982]. One of the major consequences of higher levels of impairment is activity restrictions [Duke-Elder and Abrams, 1970; Sherman, 1972; Post, 1978]. Because any deficiency of acuity is likely to affect a child's performance, in or out of school, the general effect of impairment is an increase in stress during childhood. Impaired acuity may also have other physiologic consequences. Specifically, amblyopia may develop when refractive errors are unequal in the two eyes

[Stager, 1977]. Amblyopia reduces binocular vision to monocular vision by eliminating stereoscopic depth perception.

For a child's vision problems to have a good prognosis it is crucial that the child be treated as soon as the problems are recognized and diagnosed [Post, 1978; Taylor, 1980]. The retina and occipital cortex are incomplete at birth, and their development depends on use. If the eye has trouble receiving a stimulus, vision will be impaired because the actual apparatus for seeing will not develop fully [Gardiner, 1978]. Therefore, correction of visual disorders is far more important among children than adults, and treatment may begin as early as one year. It is worthwhile to treat children with relatively small refractive errors whenever symptoms of ocular fatigue such as irritated eyes, headaches, and tiredness are experienced.

Visual deficiencies resulting from refractive errors can be corrected through the prescription of glasses or contact lenses. Because prescription of glasses is a simple and inexpensive procedure and inflicts no risk to the patient, it is the preferred treatment for almost all children who need to improve their visual acuity.

Measurements of visual acuity were obtained for each eye separately [Rubenstein et al., 1985]. If a child could read letters, the Snellen Eye Chart was used; otherwise the Picture Eye Chart or the Illiterate E Chart was used, the preference going to the Illiterate E Chart. Vision testing was done with 300- to 500-foot lumens of light, at eye level. The room was lit with additional nonglare lighting to achieve the desired illumination. Medical assistants, trained by a board-certified ophthalmologist, conducted the examinations. If the examinee had glasses or contact lenses, both the corrected and uncorrected near and far vision were tested. For far vision testing, the examinee was asked to read the line equivalent to 20/40 with one eye occluded. If more than one letter was missed, the examinee was asked to read the next line up until only one letter on a line was missed. If the examinee successfully read the 20/40 line, testing proceeded down the chart to smaller print until the line equivalent to 20/15 was reached. In this evaluation of the effects of cost sharing we present data for children's far vision with usual correction in the better eye.

HEARING LOSS

When speech and nonspeech hearing loss rates are combined nearly 19 percent of children experience some difficulty. Most hearing loss among children is mild and likely to be temporary resulting from middle ear disease. A persistent or moderate hearing loss, however, usually has serious consequences for the child's development [Downs, 1983]. Hearing loss has been associated with speech and language learning and other learning dysfunctions. It is uncertain whether minor hearing loss as is caused by otitis media negatively affects speech or learning. Yet the number of potentially affected children is large so the issue remains of critical importance.

Kessner et al. [1974] estimated the prevalence of hearing loss among children 4 to 11 years of age. Mean threshold values were calculated for the speech frequencies (500, 1000, and 2000 Hz) and the low (125 and 250 Hz) and high (4000 and 8000 Hz) nonspeech frequencies. He found that among the 1639 children in his study, 6.7 percent experienced loss at the speech levels (2.2 percent bilateral; 4.5 percent unilateral) and 12.2 percent had a loss at the nonspeech levels (4.6 percent bilateral; 7.6 percent unilateral). The prevalence of hearing loss decreased with age. An NCHS [1970b] survey between 1963 and 1965 on the hearing status of a national probability sample of 7119 children ages 6 to 11 years found, using average hearing threshold of the speech frequencies of the better ear, that the overall prevalence of hearing loss was 1.9 percent for boys and 1.5 percent for girls. Comparisons of the age-specific rates of bilateral loss at the speech frequencies (Kessner) with the same rates of hearing loss in the better ear (NCHS) show them to be very similar for children ages 6 to 11 years.

The mild hearing loss that is common in general populations typically subsides with successful treatment of middle ear disease. Therapy consists of antibiotics or surgical procedures to relieve inflammation.

Measures of hearing acuity were obtained on children 4 to 13 years of age for each ear. The child was tested (without usual correction if used was any) with a Beltone 12–0 manual pure tone threshold audiometer while seated in a soundproof booth and using the following procedure.

The child was familiarized with the test before the actual testing began. A tone of gradually increasing intensity was presented until the child acknowledged it. The actual threshold determination started with the first test tone (1000 Hz) presented at an intensity of 20 dB below that of the familiarization tone. At the point that the examinee failed to respond, the intensity was increased in 5 dB increments until the sound was heard again. The intensity was then raised another 5 dB and, after response, decreased by 15 dB. Another series of ascending presentations was begun. For HIE purposes, the threshold was defined as the lowest level at which responses occurred in at least half of the ascents, with a minimum of three responses at a single level. This procedure was repeated to determine the thresholds of the remaining frequencies (500, 2000, and 4000 Hz).

A child is defined as having hearing loss if the average hearing threshold level in the better ear is 16 dB or more. This criteria implies that a child who is counted as being hearing impaired is in fact experiencing bilateral hearing loss because the threshold in the worse ear is higher than 16 dB. This conservative definition permits greater confidence in identification of a true hearing deficit.

FLUID IN THE MIDDLE EAR

Otitis media is among the most prevalent conditions afflicting a general population of children. Otitis media or inflammation of the middle ear usually is accompanied by the accumulation of fluid in the middle ear canal. Because screening techniques permit us only to assess the amount of fluid in the middle ear we will refer to our data in this way to avoid any misunderstanding or misinterpretations given the differing diagnostic criteria and debates about otitis media.

Published reports indicate that overall prevalence of otitis media is between 15 to 20 percent of the pediatric population. In an NCHS survey of otoscopy findings, approximately 15 percent of children ages 6 to 11 had otoscopic abnormalities of the right eardrum [NCHS, 1973b]. Several community studies report similar findings. Kessner et al. [1974] using otoscopy performed by board-certified or board-eligible otolaryngologists, found among Washington, D.C., children 6 months to 11 years that 19.2 percent suffered otitis media. Among the youngest children (6 months to 3 years) the prevalence of ear disease was 27.6 percent whereas among the oldest children (age 11) only 14.4 percent suffered ear disease. Biles et al. [1980] provide data on Galveston, Texas, children ages 0 to 8 years who received care in 1975. More than a third (35 percent) of the children at risk had one episode of otitis during the year and 12 percent had two or more episodes. The risk of developing acute otitis media is highest in the first two years of life and decreases with age.

This condition can be painful and uncomfortable for the child and can result in limitations of usual activities (school days lost) and produce considerable concern among parents. Complications from acute middle ear disease are rare. The predominant problem is mild hearing loss, which usually subsides when the inflammation resolves. Chronic otitis, inflammation exceeding 3 months duration, can be associated with complications such as a perforated or scarred eardrum and necrosis or scarring of the middle ear ossicles.

Care for otitis media involves antibiotics and symptomatic medications for acute cases, whereas in nonsuppurative cases, myringotomy (incision of the ear drum) and implantation of tympanostomy tubes are also used. All cases require careful follow up to prevent potential hearing deficits that could cause speech or learning dysfunction.

This disorder is among the most common diagnosis made by physicians for office visits by persons under 22 years of age. NCHS [1981] reports that in 1977–1978 more than 11 million visits were made to office-based physicians by patients under 15 years of age with earache or ear infection as the principal reason for visit. These visits represented over 5 percent of all visits for children under 15. NCHS [1983] reported that in 1980, 11.7 million visits were for supportative and unspecified otitis media; 77 percent were described as an acute problem, 10 percent as a flare-up of a chronic problem, and 8 percent as a routine chronic problem. Teele et al. [1983] reported that of Boston children followed in a longitudinal study for the first five years of life, the proportion of visits involving otitis ranged from about 23 percent (children under 1 year) to about 42 percent (children age 4). They found no difference in the prevalence of this disease among children from low and high socioeconomic backgrounds.

Although a clinical assessment using otoscopy rather than tympanometry would have been preferable, it was not possible given the financial constraints of the HIE. Thus, the classification of children with fluid in the middle ear is based solely on tympanometry data. Because of the limitations of these data a conservative definition was employed in the identification of children with middle ear disease.

Measurements of eardrum compliance were obtained from children ages 4 through 13 for each ear separately with an American Electronics Impedance Audiometer Modes 81 [Lohr et al., 1983]. A technician recorded the maximum compliance and the air pressure at which maximum compliance occurred. The technician also evaluated the shape of the tympanogram according to four standard "slopes."

PARENTAL WORRY

Parents were asked to describe the level of worry they experienced because of their children's health. The worry scale ranged from 1 (not at all worried) to 4 (worried a great deal).

PHYSICAL HEALTH

Our physical health measures examine limitations in the performance of various specific daily activities [Eisen et al., 1980]. Assessments of limitations were made by parental responses to a battery of questions about self-care, mobility, and physical activities.

Questionnaire items were adapted from those used for adults (14 years old and older) in the HIE [Stewart et al., 1978]. Those measures were based on the work of Patrick, Bush, and Chen [1973] and of Reynolds, Rushing, and Miles [1974], who examined functional limitations of both children and adults.

In this Note we present the effects of insurance on one aspect of physical health—role limitations—which encompass limitations on play, school, or other usual activities in any degree.

MENTAL HEALTH PERCEPTIONS

Mental health measures were designed to assess both positive and negative states of psychological well-being. As with the other health perceptions measures, assessments were based on parental responses (for children younger than 14) and self reports (for those 14 years and older) to a battery of self-administered questions. Because we followed a cohort of children 0–13 years of age at enrollment, some children were 18 years old upon exit from the study. Thus, both parental and self-reports were used in these analyses. In the HIE we examine children's mental health status through the use of the Mental Health Rating Index, which provides an aggregate assessment of the child's affective mental health (psychological distress and psychological well-being).

Questionnaire items selected for this assessment were based on content analysis of mental health survey measures of general populations and on the battery of items used for adults in the HIE [Ware et al., 1979]. The items chosen to measure mental health evaluated constructs of distress (e.g., child seemed relaxed, bothered by nervousness, anxious, worried, seemed lonely, depressed) and positive well-being (e.g., seemed cheerful or happy and enjoyed things) during the month before the questionnaire administration [Eisen et al, 1980]. Both positively and negatively worded items were used to achieve a wide range of scores and a balanced scale.

GENERAL HEALTH PERCEPTIONS

Finally, self-ratings of general health, which are among the most commonly used measures of health status, were assessed. For example, ratings of health as "excellent," "good," "fair," or "poor" have been used in the National Health Examination Survey and other health surveys. These general health measures do not assess a specific health status attribute, but they have been shown empirically to be related to a wide range of physical and mental health concepts and illness behaviors. The General Health Rating Index was used in the HIE to assess perceptions of the child's health, past, present, and future.

General health questionnaire items originally constructed for adults [Ware and Karmos, 1976] and items used in the National Health Examination Survey [NCHS, 1973b] were adapted for assessing the health of children in the HIE. Items were defined with respect to time (perceptions of prior and current general health) and with respect to resistance or susceptibility to illness. Positively and negatively worded items were used to balance the rating scale.

Appendix B

ESTIMATED REGRESSION EQUATIONS

INTRODUCTION

This appendix presents detailed information about the regression equations used to evaluate the effects of cost sharing for various measures of child health. The first subsection defines all the explanatory variables and interactions. The second section provides the estimated equations and other information about the equations.

VARIABLES USED IN REGRESSION EQUATIONS

Table B.1 defines the names of the variables used in the regression analyses. Unless otherwise noted, dummy variables are scored 1 if "yes" and 0 otherwise. Exit health status values by plan are presented in Table B.2.

RESULTS OF REGRESSION ANALYSES

We used standard linear regression models for estimating effects on General Health Ratings, Mental Health Ratings, Functional Far Vision, and Parental Worry. With the exception of vision, a higher score means better health. For the other health status measures (role limitations, anemia, hay fever, hearing loss, and fluid in the middle ear), we used maximum likelihood logit regression models. A high value on these measures indicated the presence of the condition and thus worse health. The General Health Ratings Index and Mental Health Rating Index were transformed from a standardized 0 to 100 point scale to a 0 to 10 point scale to correct for heteroskedasticity. The 0 to 100 point scale was transformed as follows:

$$X' = 10 - \sqrt{100-X} \qquad X = 0\text{--}100 \text{ scale}$$

$$X' = 0\text{--}10 \text{ scale}$$

In the remainder of this appendix detailed results of the regression analyses are presented. The standard errors and the t-tests were computed using Huber's (1967) formula for the variance of a robust regression. To apply Huber's formula, the family was considered the unit of observation and linear regression on individuals as an M-

Table B.1

GLOSSARY OF ACRONYMS

DEMOGRAPHIC

MALE	Dummy variable indicating whether the child was male (1 if male, 0 if female)
TINC	Family income as measured at baseline (three to nine months before enrollment). This value was computed by (1) standardizing the family's reported income for the two years before baseline to 1974 dollars using cost-of-living adjustments, (2) correcting for intersite differences in cost of living, (3) adding $1000, (4) dividing by a family size adjustment factor, and (5) taking the natural logarithm of this value. In all interactions, income is measure in its log form centered at its mean.
LFAMSIZE	Family size taken to the natural logarithm
NONWHITE	Dummy variable indicating race of child (1 if nonwhite; 0 if white)
AGE	Age of the child at enrollment
LESSHS	Dummy variable for parental education level less than high school
SOMECOL	Dummy variable for parental education (1 if some college; 0 otherwise)
COLLG	Dummy variable for parental education (1 if college graduate or more; 0 otherwise)
EDUC	Parental education—years of schooling

EXPERIMENTAL

TERM3	Dummy variable indicating whether child participated for three years (1 if three years; 0 if five)
INCXCOIN	Interaction between centered TINC and COSTSHARING plans
TOOKPHYS	A dummy variable indicating whether child took medical screening examination at enrollment
HRTYPE	A dummy variable indicating whether health diary was kept during participation
COINS	Dummy variable indicating child was assigned to the 25% or 95% cost-sharing plan
FREE	Dummy variable indicating whether child was assigned to the 0% cost-sharing fee-for-service plan
GHE	Dummy variable indicating whether the child was assigned to care under the Group Health Cooperative by the experiment
GHC	Dummy variable indicating whether the child was a member of Group Health Cooperative participating in our control group

HEALTH STATUS MEASURES

ROLEDUM4	Dummy variable indicates enrollment response on infant (0–4) form of medical history
ROLEDUM6	Dummy variable indicates enrollment response on adult (14+) form of medical history
ROLE0	Enrollment role limitations (1 if limited; 0 otherwise)
ROLEX	Exit role limitations (1 if limited; 0 otherwise)

Table B.1—continued

DUM1X4	Dummy variable indicates pediatric (5–13) form responses at enrollment and exit
SQRMHI0	Enrollment Mental Health Rating Index; 0–10 scale, higher score better mental health
SQRMHIX	Exit Mental Health Rating Index; 0–10 scale, higher score better mental health
DUM1X4	Dummy variable indicates infant form response at enrollment and exit
DUM1X5	Dummy variable indicates infant form response at enrollment and pediatric at exit
DUM2X5	Dummy variable indicates pediatric form response at enrollment and exit
SQRGHI0	Enrollment General Health Rating Index; 0–10 scale, higher score better health
SQRGHIX	Exit General Health Rating Index; 0–10 scale, higher score better health
BINSTAT	Dummy variable of hemoglobin status at enrollment (1 if low hemoglobin; 0 otherwise)
BINSTATX	Dummy variable of hemoglobin status at exit (1 if low hemoglobin; 0 otherwise)
HAYFCURT	Dummy variable of bothered by hay fever and other plant allergies at enrollment (1 if bothered; 0 otherwise)
HAYCURTX	Dummy variable of bothered by hay fever and other plant allergies at exit (1 if bothered; 0 otherwise)
BIN1HEAR	Dummy variable of hearing impairment at enrollment (1 if impaired; 0 otherwise)
BIN1HERX	Dummy variable of hearing impairment at exit (1 if impaired; 0 otherwise)
BIN30TMD	Dummy variable of fluid in middle ear at enrollment (1 if fluid; 0 otherwise)
BIN30TMX	Dummy variable of fluid in middle ear at exit (1 if fluid; 0 otherwise)
BLINFUNF	Far vision in Snellen lines at enrollment
BLINFUNFX	Far vision in Snellen lines at exit
WORRY0	Parental worry about health in general at enrollment; scale 1–4, higher score more worry
WORRYX	Parental worry about health in general at exit; scale 1–4, higher score more worry
SQRREL0	Enrollment Social Relations index; 0–10 scale, higher score better social health
SQRRELX	Exit Social Relations index; 0–10 scale, higher score better social health
POLIOB00	
TETBOOS0	

estimator. (An M-estimator is a type of robust estimator.) Linear regression is not the maximum likelihood estimator because individuals within a family have correlated responses. By calculating $R_2 R_1 R_2$, which is an asymptotically consistent estimate of the covariance matrix of the regression parameters, we correct for the intrafamily correlation regardless of its form or heteroskedasticity.

R_1 and R_2 are defined as follows:

$$R_1 = \sum_{\text{across families}} (\sum_{\text{within family}} X_i r_i)' (\sum_{\text{within family}} X_i r_i)$$

$$R_2 = (X'X)^{-1} \sigma^2 .$$

X_i represents the matrix of observed data and r_i the vector of residuals for family member i.

Table B.2

HEALTH STATUS VALUES OF CHILDREN AGED 3 TO 18 YEARS
UPON COMPLETION OF EXPERIMENTAL PARTICIPATION
BY INSURANCE PLAN TYPE[a]

| | Fee-For-Service | | | | Prepaid Group Practice | | | |
| | Copay | | Free | | Experimental | | Control | |
Health Status Measure[a]	N	Mean (s.e.)	N	Mean (s.e.)	N	Mean (s.e.)	N	Mean (s.e.)
Role limitations(%)	189	3.7	117	3.1	303	2.9	120	3.1
Social relations[c]	164	74.9 (1.67)	99	75.4 (2.23)	268	76.4 (1.22)	117	75.8 (1.94)
Behavior problems[d]	123	15.7 (0.72)	71	16.2 (0.87)	187	17.0 (0.62)	79	17.7 (0.99)
Mental health[c]	167	5.9 (0.11)	100	5.8 (0.13)	269	5.7 (0.09)	117	5.8 (0.14)
General health[c]	187	6.0 (0.15)	117	5.8 (0.17)	303	5.4 (0.10)	120	5.5 (0.17)
Anemia(%)	178	3.4	108	1.0	274	1.0	114	1.0
Hay Fever(%)	130	20.8	83	19.3	206	20.4	88	21.6
Vision, corrected[e]	180	2.9 (0.10)	106	2.4 (0.09)	287	2.7 (0.08)	114	3.1 (0.15)
Hearing loss(%)	164	9.8	91	11.0	255	7.1	116	7.8
Fluid in middle ear(%)	125	36.0	61	41.0	169	27.2	69	14.5
Polio booster(%)	122	10.7	69	4.3	187	5.9	77	2.6
Tetanus booster(%)	122	8.2	69	10.1	186	6.5	77	3.9
Parental worry[f]	145	1.6 (0.06)	88	1.4 (0.07)	221	1.6 (0.05)	82	1.5 (0.07)

[a]Insurance plans: fee-for-service—25 percent and 95 percent coinsurance plans (copay), 0 percent coinsurance plan (free); prepaid group practice—experimentals (GHE) and controls (GHC). The control group is self-selected.

[b]Sample sizes across measures are dissimilar because the number of children included in each health status analysis differs because of age restrictions or missing data.

[c]0–10 scale; a higher value denotes better health.

[d]0–100 scale; a higher value denotes poorer health.

[e]In Snellen line values: 2 = 20/20, 3 = 20/25, 4 = 20/30.

[f]Four-point scale: 4 = a great deal, 3 = somewhat, 2 = a little, 1 = not at all.

Table B.3

ESTIMATED REGRESSION MODEL AND CORRECTED t-TEST VALUES: ROLE LIMITATIONS

Variable	Logit Coefficient	t-Test
INTERCEPT	−3.63	−7.20
ROLEDUM4	0.88	1.43
ROLEDUM6	0.11	0.21
MALE	−0.32	−0.72
FREE	−0.08	−0.12
GHE	−0.38	−0.70
GHC	0.03	0.05
ROLELIMO	2.83	5.50

N = 729
Chi-Squared = 24.39
Log Likelihood Ratio = 12.20

Table B.4

ESTIMATED REGRESSION MODEL AND CORRECTED t-TEST VALUES: SOCIAL RELATIONS

Variable	Coefficient	t-Test
INTERCEPT	10.43	3.34
SQRREL0	0.38	4.87
AGE	−0.19	−6.53
MALE	0.11	0.73
TINC	−0.40	−1.21
INCXFREE	0.64	1.31
INCXGHE	0.74	1.76
INCXGHC	0.44	0.64
FREE	0.10	0.41
GHE	0.29	1.49
GHC	0.03	0.09

N = 448
Est. Std. Dev. = 1.603
R-Squared = 0.1542

Table B.5

ESTIMATED REGRESSION MODEL AND CORRECTED t-TEST VALUES: BEHAVIOR PROBLEMS

Variable	Coefficient	t-Test
INTERCEPT	42.96	2.33
SQRMHIO	−2.20	−6.10
AGE	0.21	0.75
MALE	0.74	0.77
TINC	−1.74	−0.89
INCXFREE	1.35	0.48
INCXGHE	2.32	0.93
INCXGHC	1.48	0.34
FREE	1.38	0.89
GHE	1.96	1.71
GHC	1.21	0.73

N = 269
R-Squared = 7.632
Est. Std. Dev. = 0.1428

Table B.6

ESTIMATED REGRESSION MODEL AND CORRECTED t-TEST VALUES: MENTAL HEALTH

Variable	Coefficient	t-Test
INTERCEPT	11.64	3.93
SQRMHI0	0.42	7.98
DUM1X3	0.24	0.94
LFAMSIZE	−0.27	−0.99
NONWHITE	−0.51	−1.58
AGE	−0.04	−0.76
EDUC	−0.02	−0.64
TOOKPHYS	0.06	0.42
MALE	−0.05	−0.37
TINC	−0.80	−2.58
INCXFREE	1.10	2.42
INCXGHE	1.02	2.60
INCXGHC	0.63	0.99
FREE	−0.07	−0.30
GHE	−0.19	−1.06
GHC	−0.13	−0.48

N = 449
Est. Std. Dev. = 1.2697
R squared = 0.2164

Table B.7

ESTIMATED REGRESSION MODEL AND CORRECTED
t-TEST VALUES: GENERAL HEALTH

Variable	Coefficient	t-Test
INTERCEPT	5.14	1.72
SQRGHI0	0.40	11.25
DUM1X4	−0.76	−1.80
DUM1X5	−0.17	−0.57
DUM2X6	−0.90	−3.07
LFAMSIZE	0.41	1.44
NONWHITE	−0.23	−0.70
AGE	−0.06	−1.05
LESSHS	0.23	1.05
SOMECOL	0.07	0.36
COLLG	0.06	0.30
TOOKPHYS	−0.07	−0.49
MALE	−0.02	−0.11
TINC	−0.17	−0.53
INCXFREE	0.62	1.43
INCXGHE	0.38	0.98
INCXGHC	0.76	1.36
FREE	−0.05	−0.21
GHE	−0.41	−2.28
GHC	−0.28	−1.10

N = 684
Est. St. Dev. = 1.645
R-squared = 0.2579
t-tests deflated by 1.1233 for intrafamily correlation

Table B.8

ESTIMATED REGRESSION MODEL AND CORRECTED t-TEST
VALUES: FAR VISION WITH USUAL CORRECTION

Variable	Coefficient	t-Test
INTERCEPT	4.32	4.46
BLINFUNF	0.07	2.26
AGE	−0.14	−10.46
TINC	−0.07	−0.62
MALE	−0.03	−0.33
FREE	−0.46	−3.01
GHE	−0.17	−1.47
GHC	0.25	1.67

N = 687
Est. Std. Dev. = 1.231
R-Squared = 0.1700

Table B.9

ESTIMATED REGRESSION MODEL AND CORRECTED t-TEST VALUES: HEARING LOSS

Variable	Logit Coefficient	t-Test
INTERCEPT	5.91	1.23
TINC	−0.93	−1.79
INCXFREE	1.26	1.58
INCXGHE	0.49	0.69
INCXGHC	0.03	0.03
FREE	0.28	0.62
GHE	−0.29	−0.75
GHC	−0.11	−0.23
BIN1HEAR	−1.08	−2.53

N = 626
Chi-Squared = 16.82
Log Likelihood Ratio = 8.41

Table B.10

ESTIMATED REGRESSION MODEL AND CORRECTED t-TEST VALUES: FLUID IN MIDDLE EAR

Variable	Logit Coefficient	t-Test
INTERCEPT	−0.52	−0.13
AGE	−0.13	−2.52
MALE	−0.02	−0.07
TINC	0.08	0.19
INCXFREE	−0.37	−0.61
INCXGHE	−0.22	−0.39
INCXGHC	−0.005	−0.01
FREE	0.14	0.41
GHE	−0.47	−1.81
GHC	−1.32	−3.14
BIN3OTMD	0.22	0.81

N = 424
Chi-Squared = 24.04
Log Likelihood Ratio = 12.02

Table B.11

ESTIMATED REGRESSION MODEL AND CORRECTED
t-TEST VALUES: ANEMIA

Variable	Logit Coefficient	t-Test
INTERCEPT	5.35	1.04
TINC	−0.93	−1.67
FREE	−1.42	−1.31
GHE	−1.52	−1.89
GHC	−1.08	−0.99
BINSTAT	0.78	0.87

N = 674
Chi-Squared = 8.01
Log Likelihood Ratio = 4.003

Table B.12

ESTIMATED REGRESSION MODEL AND CORRECTED
t-TEST VALUES: HAY FEVER

Variable	Logit Coefficient	t-Test
INTERCEPT	−9.49	−1.49
GHC	−0.15	−0.33
GHE	0.08	0.26
FREE	−0.06	−0.16
INCXFREE	0.11	0.12
INCXGHE	0.13	0.15
INCXGHC	−0.85	−0.70
TINC	0.70	1.04
AGE	0.17	3.77
HAYFCURT	2.05	5.78

N = 507
Chi-Squared = 96.69
Log Likelihood Ratio = 48.35

Table B.13

ESTIMATED REGRESSION MODEL AND CORRECTED
t-TEST VALUES: POLIO BOOSTER

Variable	Logit Coefficient	t-Test
INTERCEPT	−11.66	−0.98
POLIOBOO	2.28	3.39
MALE	−0.62	−1.01
TINC	0.92	0.73
INCXFREE	−1.96	−1.23
INCXGHE	−1.04	−0.60
INCXGHC	1.08	0.36
FREE	0.10	0.11
GHE	−0.57	−0.79
GHC	−0.67	−0.44

N = 262
Chi-Squared = 15.28
Log Likelihood Ratio = 7.64

Table B.14

ESTIMATED REGRESSION MODEL AND CORRECTED
t-TEST VALUES: TETANUS BOOSTER

Variable	Logit Coefficient	t-Test
INTERCEPT	5.65	0.78
TETBOOS0	1.32	2.09
MALE	−0.56	−0.98
TINC	−0.92	−1.16
INCXFREE	0.72	0.64
INCXGHE	1.32	0.92
INCXGHC	3.23	1.15
FREE	1.06	1.43
GHE	−0.44	−0.60
GHC	−1.13	−0.76

N = 263
Chi-Squared = 12.50
Log Likelihood Ratio = 6.25

Table B.15

ESTIMATED REGRESSION MODEL AND CORRECTED
t-TEST VALUES: PARENTAL WORRY

Variable	Coefficient	t-test
INTERCEPT	2.59	3.66
WORRY0	0.20	4.47
AGE	0.02	1.93
MALE	0.05	0.72
TINC	−0.0002	−0.003
FREE	0.21	1.83
GHE	−0.01	−0.16
GHC	0.19	1.60

N = 509
Est Std Dev = 0.7165
R-Squared = 0.0827
Parental Worry variable is scored 1 = A Great Deal
4 = Not at all

BIBLIOGRAPHY

Beck S., K. N. Lohr, C. J. Kamberg, et al., *Measurement of Physiologic Health for Children: Vol. 1, Allergic Conditions*, The RAND Corporation, R-2898/1-HHS, January 1983.

Biles, R. W., P. A. Buffler, and A. A. O'Donell, "Epidemiology of Otitis Media: A Community Study," *American Journal of Public Health*, Vol. 70, 1980, pp. 593–598.

Broder, I., M. W. Higgins, K. A. Matthews, et al., "Epidemiology of Asthma and Allergic Rhinitis in a Total Community, Tecumseh, Michigan, III. Second Survey of the Community," *The Journal of Allergy and Clinical Immunology*, Vol. 53, 1974, pp. 127–138.

Brook, R. H., J. E. Ware, A. Davies-Avery, et al., "Overview of Adult Health Status Measures Fielded in RAND's Health Insurance Study," *Medical Care*, Vol. 17, No. 7, 1979, pp. 1–131.

Brook, R. H., J. E. Ware, Jr., W. H. Rogers, et al., *The Effect of Coinsurance on the Health of Adults: Results from the RAND Health Insurance Experiment*, The RAND Corporation, R-3055-HHS, December 1984.

CDC, "Nutrition Surveillance—United States, 1980," *Mortality and Morbidity Weekly Report*, Vol. 30, No. 41, 1981, pp. 521–524.

Dacie, J. V., and S. M. Lewis, *Practical Hematology*, 5th Edition, Churchill Livingstone, Edinburgh, 1975.

Dagenais, M. G., "Further Suggestions Concerning the Utilization of Incomplete Observations in Regression Analysis," *Journal of the American Statistics Association*, Vol. 66, 1971, pp. 93–98.

Dallman, P. R., "Iron Deficiency: Diagnosis and Treatment (Nutrition in Medicine)," *Western Journal of Medicine*, Vol. 134, 1981, pp. 496–505.

Davies, A. R., et al., "Consumer Acceptance of Prepaid and Fee-for Service Medical Care: Results from a Randomized Trial," *Health Services Research*, Vol. 21, August 1986, pp. 429–452.

Diehr, P. K., W. C. Richardson, S. M. Shortell, J. P. LoGerfo, "Increased Access to Medical Care: The Impact on Health," *Medical Care*, Vol. 17, No. 10, 1979, pp. 989–999.

Downs, M., "An Audiologist's Overview of the Sequelae of Early Otitis Media: Workshop on Effects of Otitis Media on the Child," *Pediatrics*, Vol. 71, 1983, pp. 643–644.

Duke-Elder, W. S., and D. Abrams, "Ophthalmic Optics and Refraction," in W. S. Duke-Elder (ed.), *Systems of Ophthalmology*, Vol. 5, C.V. Mosby Company, St. Louis, 1970.

Dutton, D. B., "Hematocrit Levels and Race: An Argument Against the Adoption of Separate Standards in Screening for America," *Journal of the National Medical*

Association, Vol. 71, 1979, pp. 945–954.

Dutton, D. B., and R. S. Silber, "Children's Health Outcomes in Six Different Ambulatory Care Delivery Systems," *Medical Care*, Vol. 18, No. 7, 1980, pp. 693–713.

Eisen, M., C. A. Donald, J. E. Ware, et al., *Conceptualization and Measurement of Health for Children in the Health Insurance Study*, The RAND Corporation, R-2313-HEW, May 1980.

Falkson, J. L., *HMOs and the Politics of Health System Reform*, Robert J. Brady Co., New York, 1980.

Foxman B., K. N. Lohr, and R. H. Brook, *Measurement of Physiologic Health for Children: Volume 5: Anemia*, The RAND Corporation, R-2898/5-HHS, January 1983.

Gardiner, P. A., "ABC of Ophthalmology: Management of Defects of Vision in Early Childhood," *British Medical Journal*, Vol. 2, 1978, pp. 1411–1413.

Goldberg, G. A., *The Health Insurance Experiment's Guidelines for Abstracting Health Services Rendered by Group Health Cooperative of Puget Sound*, The RAND Corporation, N-1948-HHS, February 1983.

Hoekelman, R. A., M. Klein, J. E. Strain, "Who Should Provide Primary Health Care to Children: Pediatricians or Family Medicine Physicians?" *Pediatrics*, Vol. 74, No. 3, 1984, pp. 460–477.

Huber, P. J., *The Behavior or Maximum Likelihood Estimates under Nonstandard Conditions*, Fifth Berkeley Symposium, 1965, University of California Press, Berkeley, 1967, pp. 221–233.

Interstudy, National HMO Census 1985, Excelsior, Minnesota, 1986.

Kessner D. M., C. K. Snow, and J. Singer, *Assessment of Medical Care for Children: Contrasts in Health Status*, Vol. 3, Washington, D.C., Institute of Medicine, National Academy of Sciences, 1974.

Kessner, D. M., and C. E. Kalk, *A Strategy for Evaluating Health Status*, Vol. 2, Institute of Medicine, National Academy of Sciences, Washington, D.C., 1973, pp. 96–118.

Lanzkowsky, M. D., "Iron Deficiency Anemia," *Pediatrics Annals*, Vol. 3, No. 3, 1974, pp. 6–33.

Leibowitz, A., W. G. Manning, E. B. Keeler, et al., "The Effect of Cost Sharing on the Use of Medical Services by Children: Interim Results from a Randomized Controlled Trial," *Pediatrics*, Vol. 75, No. 5, 1985, pp. 942–951.

Lohr, K. N., S. Beck, C. Kamberg, et al., *Measurement of Physiologic Health for Children: Volume 2: Middle Ear Disease and Hearing Impairment*, The RAND Corporation, R-2898/2-HHS, October 1983.

MacColl, W. A., *Group Practice and Prepayment of Medical Care*, Public Affairs Press, Washington, D.C., 1966.

Manning, W. G., A. Leibowitz, G. A. Goldberg, et al., "A Controlled Trial of the Effect of a Prepaid Group Practice on the Utilization of Services," *New England Journal of Medicine*, Vol. 310, 1984, pp. 1505–1510.

Manning, W. G., A. Leibowitz, G. A. Goldberg, et al., *A Controlled Trial of the Effect of a Prepaid Group Practice on the Utilization of Medical Services*, The RAND Corporation, R-3029-HHS, September 1985.

Manning, W. G., K. B. Wells, and B. Benjamin, *Use of Outpatient Mental Health Care: Trial of a Prepaid Group Practice Versus Fee-for-Service*, The RAND Corporation, R-3277-NIMH, August 1986.

Marquis, M. S., *Cost-Sharing and the Patient's Choice of Provider*, The RAND Corporation, R-3126-HHS, September 1984.

Morris, C. N., "A Finite Selection Model for Experimental Design of the Health Insurance Study," *Journal of Econometrics*, Vol. 11, 1979, pp. 43–61.

National Center for Health Statistics (NCHS), *Visual Acuity of Children, United States*, DHEW Publication No. 1000, Series 11, No. 101, Department of Health, Education, and Welfare, Rockville, Maryland, February 1970a.

National Center for Health Statistics (NCHS), *Hearing Levels of Children by Age and Sex, United States*, Series 11, No. 102, U. S. Department of Health, Education, and Welfare, Washington, D.C., 1970b.

National Center for Health Statistics (NCHS), *Prevalence of Selected Chronic Respiratory Conditions, United States, 1970*, DHEW Publication No. (HRA) 74-1511, Series 10, No. 84, Department of Health, Education, and Welfare, Health Resources Administration, Rockville, Maryland, 1973a.

National Center for Health Statistics (NCHS), *Examination and Health History Findings Among Children and Youths, 6–17, United States, 1963–1970*, DHEW Publication No. (HRA) 74-1611, Series 11, No. 129, Department of Health, Education, and Welfare, Health Resources Administration, Rockville, Maryland, 1973b.

National Center for Health Statistics (NCHS), *Refraction Status of Youths 12–17 Years, United States*, DHEW Publication No. (HRA) 75–1630, Series 11, No. 148, Department of Health, Education, and Welfare, Rockville, Maryland, December 1974.

National Center for Health Statistics (NCHS), *Monocular Visual Acuity of Persons 4–74 Years, United States, 1971–1972*, DHEW Publication No. (HRA) 77-1646, Series 11, No. 201, Department of Health, Education, and Welfare, Rockville, Maryland, March 1977.

National Center for Health Statistics (NCHS), *The National Ambulatory Medical Care Survey, 1977 Summary, United States, January-December 1977*, DHEW Publication No. (PHS) 80-1795, Series 13, No. 44, Department of Health, Education, and Welfare, Hyattsville, Maryland, 1980.

National Center for Health Statistics (NCHS), *Patients' Reasons for Visiting Physicians: National Ambulatory Medical Care Survey, United States, 1977–78*, DHHS Publication No. (PHS) 82-1717, Series 13, No. 56, U.S. Department of Health and Human Services, Hyattsville, Maryland, 1981.

National Center for Health Statistics (NCHS), *Medication Therapy in Office Visits for Selected Diagnoses: The National Ambulatory Medical Care Survey: United States, 1980*, DHHS Publication No. (PHS) 83-1732, Series 13, No. 71, U.S. Department of Health and Human Services, Hyattsville, Maryland, 1983.

National Society for the Prevention of Blindness (NSPB), "Children's Eye Health Guide," NSPB, Inc., New York, March 1982.

Newhouse, J. P., "A Design for a Health Insurance Experiment," *Inquiry*, Vol. 11, 1974, pp. 5–27.

Patrick, D. L., J. W. Bush, and M. M. Chen, "Toward an Operational Definition of Health," *Journal of Health and Social Behavior*, Vol. 14, 1973, pp. 6–23.

Post, S., "Commentary," *Canadian Journal of Optometry*, Vol. 40, 1978, p. 48.

Reynolds, W. J., W. A. Rushing, and D. L. Miles, "The Validation of a Function Status Index," *Journal of Health and Social Behavior*, Vol. 15, 1974, pp. 271–288.

Rubenstein, R. S., K. N. Lohr, R. H. Brook, et al., *Measurement of Physiologic Health for Children: Volume 4: Vision Impairments*, The RAND Corporation, R-2898/4-HHS, April 1985.

Rudolph, A. M. (ed.), *Pediatrics*, 16th Edition, Appleton-Century-Crofts, New York, 1977.

Sherman, A., "A Review of Visual Screening of Schoolchildren," *British Journal of Physiological Optics*, Vol. 27, 1972, pp. 29–42.

Sloss, E., E. Keeler, B. Operskalski, et al., "Effect of a Health Maintenance Organization on Physiologic Health," *Annals of Internal Medicine*, Vol. 106, 1987, pp. 130–138.

Smith, L. H., G. A. Goldberg, R. H. Brook, et al., *The Health Insurance Study Screening Examination Procedures Manual*, The RAND Corporation, R-2101-HEW, September 1978.

Smith-Staruch, K., N. Breslau, M. Weitzman, et al., "Use of Health Services by Chronically Ill and Disabled Children," *Medical Care*, Vol. 22, 1984, pp. 310–328.

Stager, D. R., "Amblyopia and the Pediatrician," *Pediatric Annals*, Vol. 6, 1977, pp. 46–75.

Stewart, A. L., J. E., Ware, Jr., R. H. Brook, and A. Davies-Avery, *Conceptualization and Measurement of Health for Adults in the Health Insurance Study, Vol. II: Physical Health in Terms of Functioning*, The RAND Corporation, R-1987/2-HEW, July 1978.

Taylor, D., "Squint: Practical Aspects of Diagnosis and Management," *The Practitioner*, Vol. 224, 1980, pp. 587–590.

Teele, D. W., S. O., Klein, B. Rosner, et al., "Middle Ear Disease and the Practice of Pediatrics: Burden During the First Five Years of Life," *Journal of the American Medical Association*, Vol. 249, 1983, pp. 1026–1029.

Valdez, R. B., *Effects of Cost Sharing on the Health of Children*, The RAND Corporation, R-3270-HHS, March 1986.

Ware, J. E., Jr., and A. H. Karmos, *Development and Validation of Scales to Measure Perceived Health and Patient Role Propensity*, Vol. II of a Final Report, Illinois University School of Medicine, Carbondale, 1976.

Ware, J. E, Jr., S. A. Johnston, A. Davies-Avery, and R. H. Brook, *Conceptualization and Measurement of Health for Adults in the Health Insurance Study, Vol. III*,

Mental Health, The RAND Corporation, R-1987/3-HEW, December 1979.

Ware, J. E., R. H. Brook, W. H. Rogers, et al., "Comparison of Health Outcomes at a Health Maintenance Organization with Those of Fee-For Service Care," *Lancet*, Vol. 1, May 1986, pp. 1017–1022.

Ware, J. E., R. H. Brook, W. H. Rogers, et al., *Health Outcomes for Adults in Prepaid and Fee-for-Service Systems of Care*, The RAND Corporation, R-3459-HHS, October 1987.

Zellner, A., "An Efficient Method of Estimating Seemingly Unrelated Regressions and Tests for Aggregation Bias," *Journal of the American Statistics Association*, Vol. 57, 1962, pp. 348–368.

DATE DUE